IMMUNIZATIONS SAVING LIVES

Rae Simons

The Kids' Guide to Disease & Wellness:
Why People Get Sick and How They Can Stay Well
IMMUNIZATIONS: SAVING LIVES

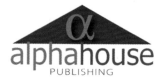

AlphaHouse Publishing
201 Harding Avenue
Vestal, NY 13850

First Printing

9 8 7 6 5 4 3 2 1

ISBN: 978-1-934970-21-8
ISBN (series): 978-1-934970-11-9
   Library of Congress Control Number: 2008930680

Author: Simons, Rae

Cover design by MK Bassett-Harvey.
Interior design by MK Bassett-Harvey and Wendy Arakawa.

Printed in India by International Print-O-Pac Limited

 An ISO 9001 Company

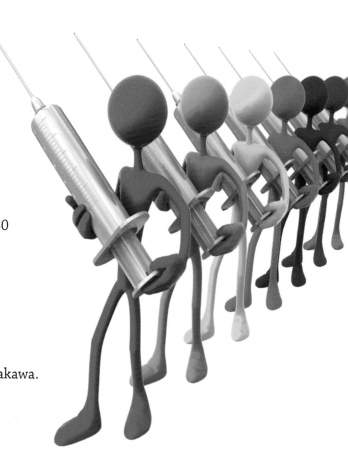

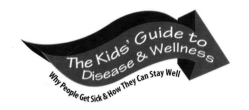

The Kids' Guide to
Disease & Wellness
Why People Get Sick & How They Can Stay Well

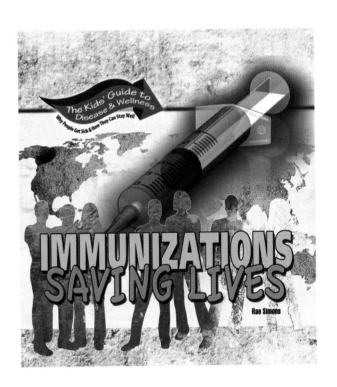

IMMUNIZATIONS
SAVING LIVES
Rae Simons

by Rae Simons

Series List

Introduction

According to a recent study reported in the Virginia Henderson International Nursing Library, kids worry about getting sick. They worry about AIDS and cancer, about allergies and the "super-germs" that resist medication. They know about these ills—but they don't always understand what causes them or how they can be prevented.

Unfortunately, most 9- to 11–year–olds, the study found, get their information about diseases like AIDS from friends and television; only 20 percent of the children interviewed based their understanding of illness on facts they had learned at school. Too often, kids believe urban legends, schoolyard folktales, and exaggerated movie plots. Oftentimes, misinformation like this only makes their worries worse. The January 2008 *Child Health News* reported that 55 percent of all children between 9 and 13 "worry almost all the time" about illness.

This series, **The Kids' Guide to Disease and Wellness**, offers readers clear information on various illnesses and conditions, as well as the immunizations that can prevent many diseases. The books dispel the myths with clearly presented facts and colorful, accurate illustrations. Better yet, these books will help kids understand not only illness—but also what they can do to stay as healthy as possible.

—*Dr. Elise Berlan*

Just The Facts

- Immunizations are small amounts of a substance put into your body so that you can fight off a disease or substance the next time it enters your body.

- People have attempted to create vaccinations throughout history. Some of the first vaccinations were developed thousands of years ago by the Chinese to fight smallpox.

- In the 1800s, germs were discovered. Later, germs from the cowpox disease were used to immunize people against smallpox.

- Polio, whooping cough, measles, mumps, tetanus, meningitis, chickenpox, the flu, and other diseases all have vaccinations to protect against them.

- Many people around the world still die from preventable diseases because they don't have access to vaccinations—especially children.

- The World Health Organization is working to bring vaccinations to kids around the world.

- Shots may hurt but will protect you from further pain in the future.

Once Upon a Time...

A hundred years ago, if you were a child growing up almost anywhere in the world, you wouldn't have had to worry about going to the doctor and getting your shots. Instead, the chances were good you would catch a serious disease (or two) by the time you were five. Illnesses like measles and whooping cough were just a part of growing up. Unfortunately, not every child DID grow up. Many of them died from these sicknesses.

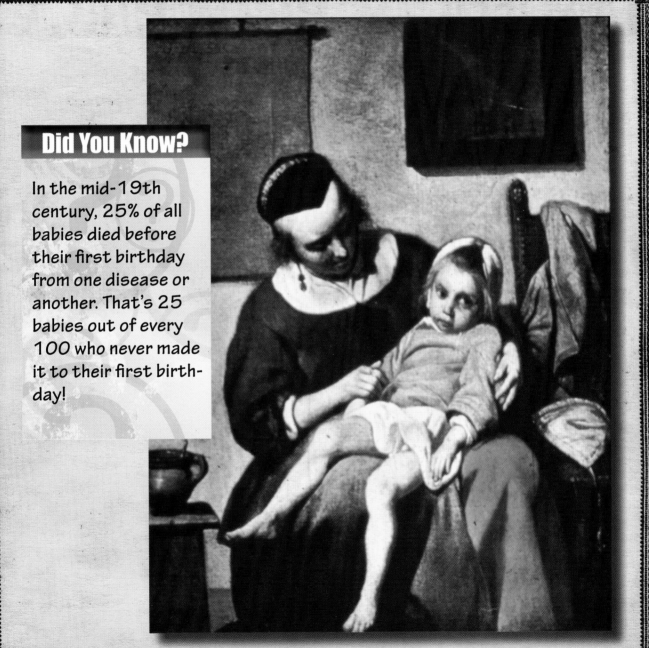

Did You Know?

In the mid-19th century, 25% of all babies died before their first birthday from one disease or another. That's 25 babies out of every 100 who never made it to their first birthday!

How Do Immunizations Work?

Nowadays, especially in the developed nations of the world, most children get shots that keep them from getting sick. These shots—also called immunizations, vaccines, or inoculations, put a little bit of some substance into your body—and that substance makes your body able to fight off a particular sickness or disease the next time it tries to invade your body. Frequently, the substance is a weak or dead germ.

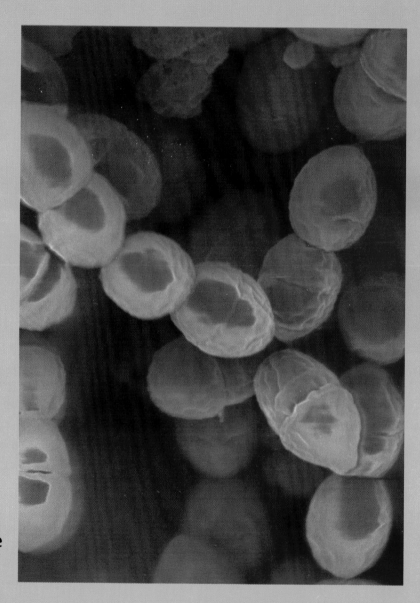

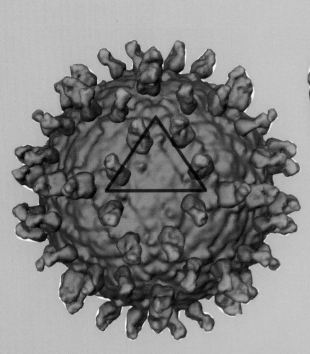

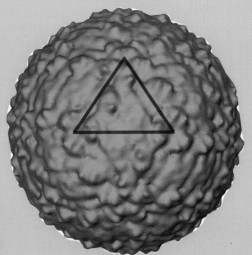

This germ doesn't make you sick—but it's enough to tell your body to create special cells called antibodies that are built to target that germ. If the germ shows up in your body, it's immediately surrounded and destroyed (as shown here).

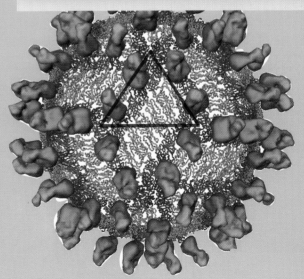

The History of Immunizations

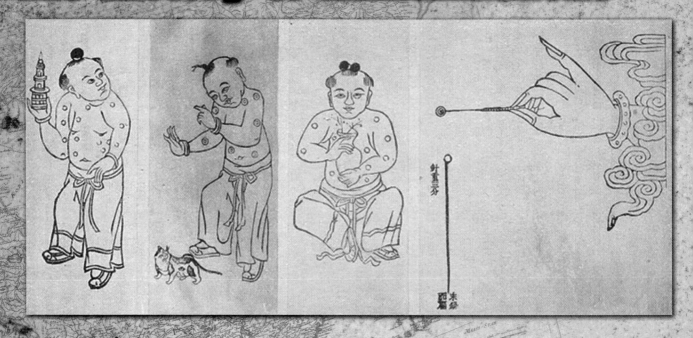

More than 2000 years ago, an ancient Chinese physician came up with the idea to put a little bit of the blood from a person with rabies or smallpox into the body of another person to keep the second person from getting sick. This practice was based on the medical belief that "like cures like." In this case, the Chinese were well ahead of the rest of the world. Physicians in Ancient Greece (right) had many wise techniques for treating sick people, but they did not know about vaccines.

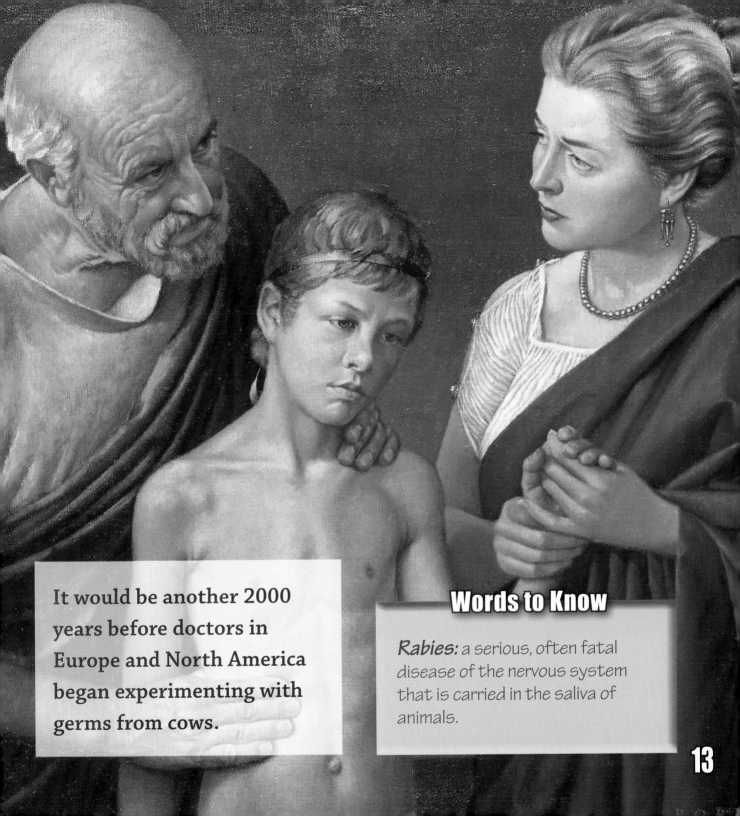

It would be another 2000 years before doctors in Europe and North America began experimenting with germs from cows.

Words to Know

Rabies: a serious, often fatal disease of the nervous system that is carried in the saliva of animals.

13

"Little Animals"

For hundreds of years, people did not understand what caused diseases. Because they didn't know about bacteria and viruses (what people often call germs), they didn't know how to keep from spreading sickness to each other. They didn't know how important clean water, clean food, and clean hands were. People dumped their toilets into the street where it flowed into drinking water and the water used for bathing and washing clothes. No one cared much about baths, let alone washing their hands before eating.

Then toward the end of the 17th century, a man named Antonie von Leeuwenhoek (shown to the right) began experimenting with very simple microscope lenses. What he saw through them amazed him: there were "tiny animals" in a drop of water! Leeuwenhoek had discovered germs.

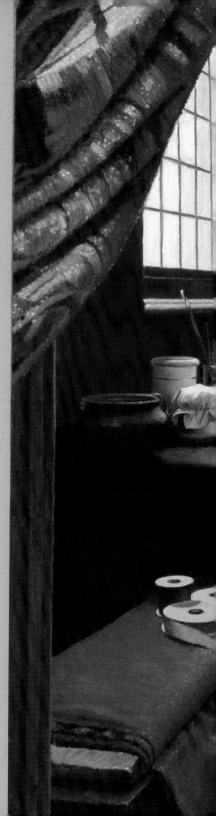

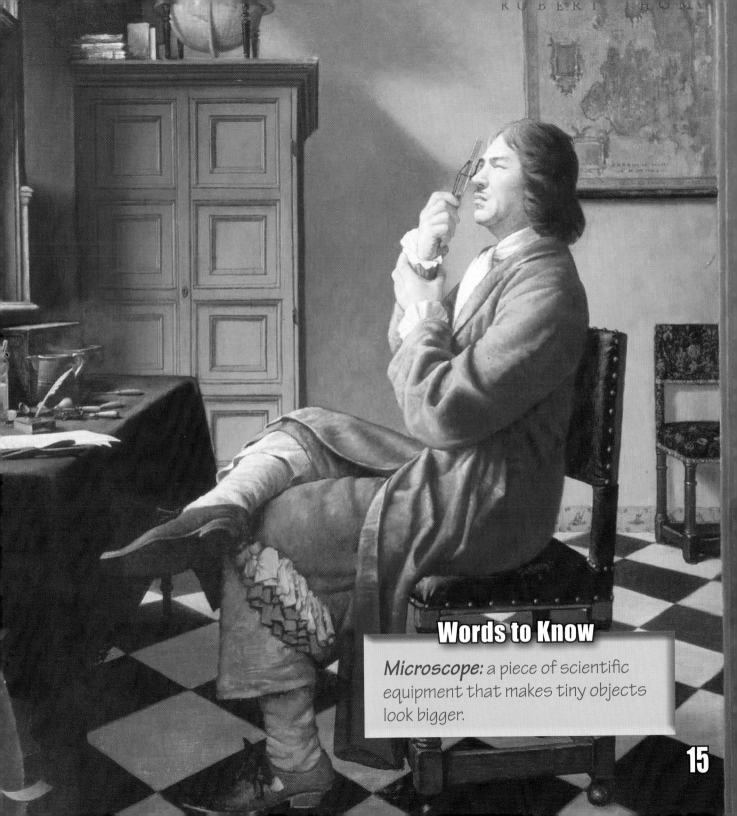

Smallpox

Smallpox was a terrible disease that made pockets of pus on people's skin. If you survived smallpox (and lots of people didn't), you would have deep scars all over you for the rest of your life. Smallpox was first discovered about 3000 years ago. It gradually spread around the world, from Africa and Asia to Europe, and from there to North and South America. Millions of people died from smallpox.

And then people began to notice something: people who got smallpox never got it again.

Words to Know

Epidemics: widespread outbreaks of a disease, affecting lots of people across a wide region.

Did You Know?

When white people first came to the Americas, they brought their germs with them, including smallpox. The native people living in the Americas had never been exposed to smallpox, and the disease swept through, killing entire tribes. Historians believe that as much as one-third of all the people in the Americas died from smallpox after their first contact with Europeans.

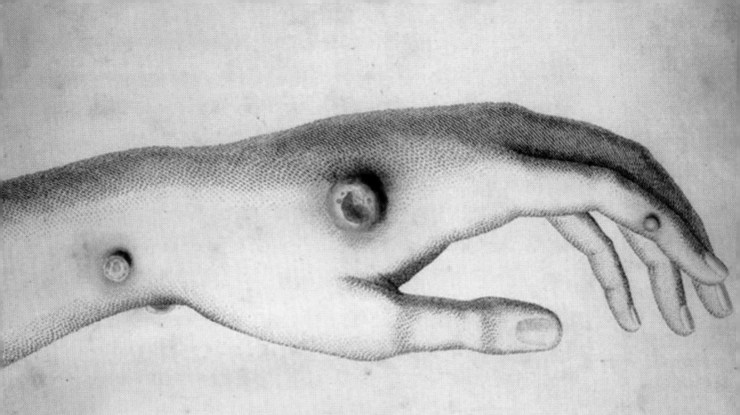

This gave people the idea of trying to give mild cases of the disease as protection against more severe cases. Sometimes people would grind up smallpox scabs and blow the powder up a person's nose. A few of these people got sick with smallpox and died. But many more only got sick a little—and from then on they were protected against the deadly disease.

Smallpox was still a big problem around the world, however. Epidemics swept through communities and countries, killing millions and millions of people.

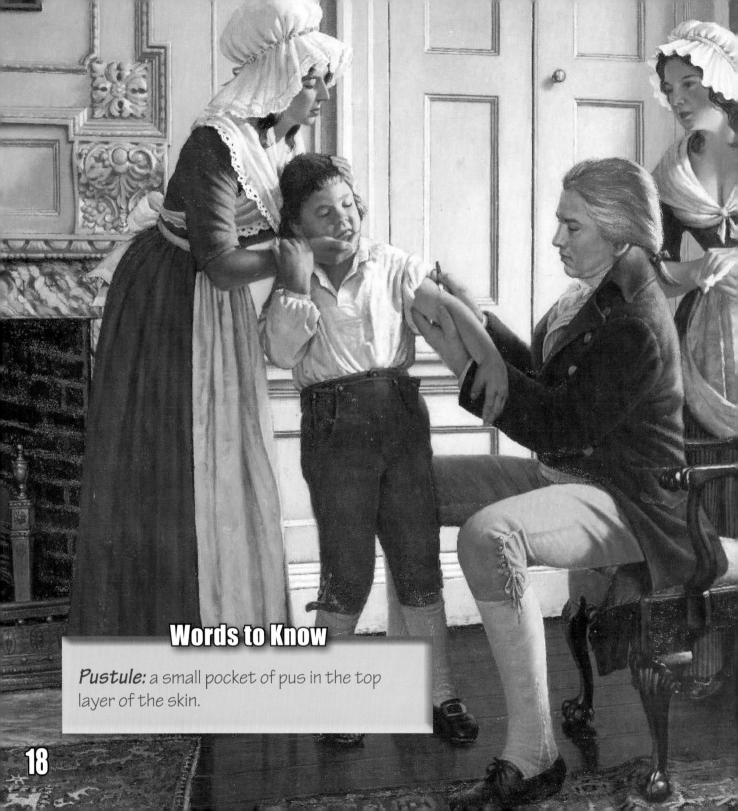

Words to Know

Pustule: a small pocket of pus in the top layer of the skin.

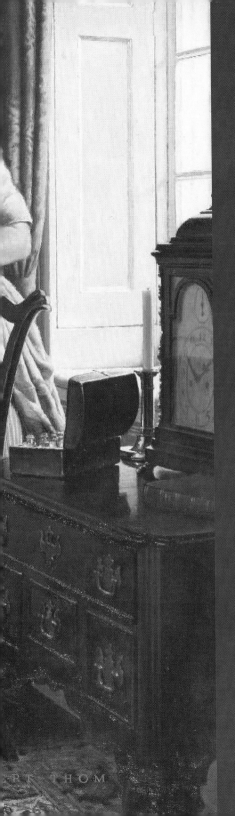

In 1796, an English doctor, Edward Jenner, noticed that milkmaids who got sick with cowpox, a less serious disease than smallpox, did not catch the more deadly disease. That gave Dr. Jenner an idea: he took the fluid from a cowpox pustule on a dairymaid's hand, scratched the skin of an 8-year-old boy, and rubbed it with the fluid. Six weeks later, he exposed the boy to smallpox. And the boy did not get sick.

At first people thought this was a crazy idea. After all, no one really liked the idea of getting scratched, let alone rubbing pus from someone else's sore onto themselves. But eventually, people began to realize that Dr. Jenner had a good idea. Once they saw that Dr. Jenner's inoculation could keep them from getting sick, the idea caught on fast. By 1800, just four years later, nearly 100,000 people had been vaccinated.

Who Was Louis Pasteur?

In the 1900s, a French chemist and biologist, Louis Pasteur, discovered more about the "tiny animals." He proved that they did not just magically appear (as people had thought), but that they were produced from other tiny creatures like themselves. He also discovered that these microscopic animals can travel through the air and that they could be killed in liquids by boiling. (The word "pasteurization," the process of killing germs in milk, comes from Pasteur's name.) As part of Pasteur's experiments, he created vaccines for rabies and anthrax.

Words to Know

Microscopic: able to be seen only through a microscope's magnifying lenses.

Anthrax: a disease that is usually caught from animals or animal products (such as wool).

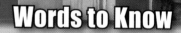

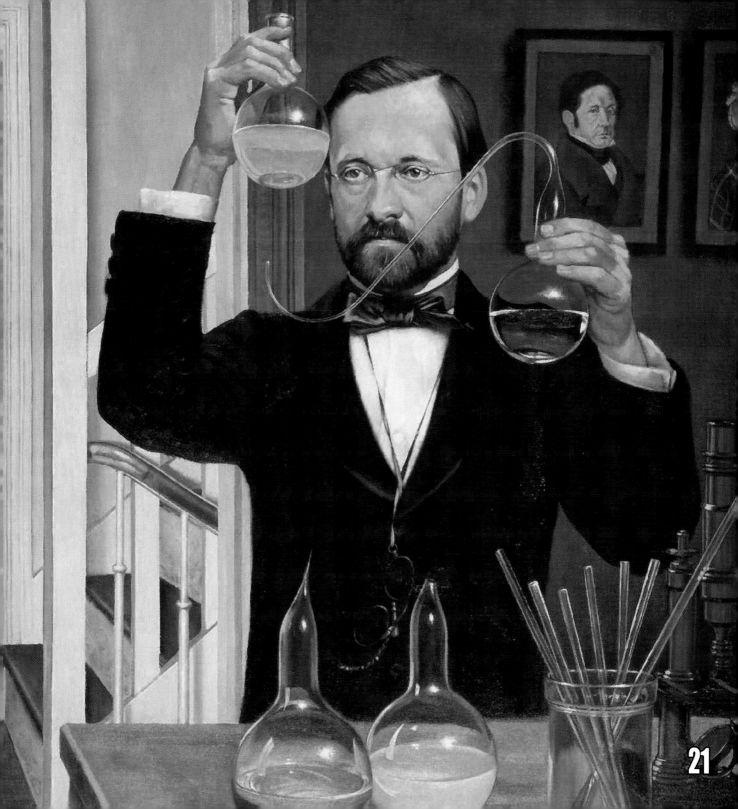

What Do Cows Have to Do With It?

The word "vaccine" comes from the Latin word for cow: "vacca."

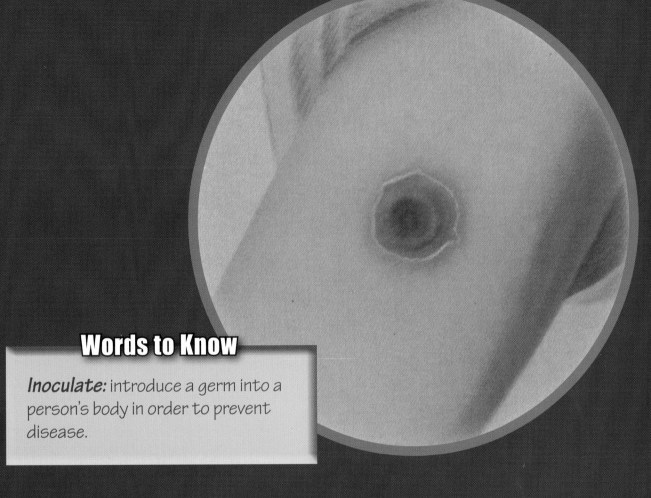

Dr. Jenner invented the word for his technique of taking pus from a cowpox pustule (shown above) to inoculate someone against smallpox. Originally, "vaccine" only referred to smallpox inoculations that came from cowpox, but gradually the word came to be used for all immunizations. So thank a cow the next time you get your shots!

What Came Next?

When Dr. Jenner vaccinated the little boy back in 1796, there was no such thing as a hypodermic needle. Children who were inoculated continued to be scratched. Fifty years later, though, the hypodermic needle was invented. This allowed doctors to inject fluid directly into people's bloodstreams.

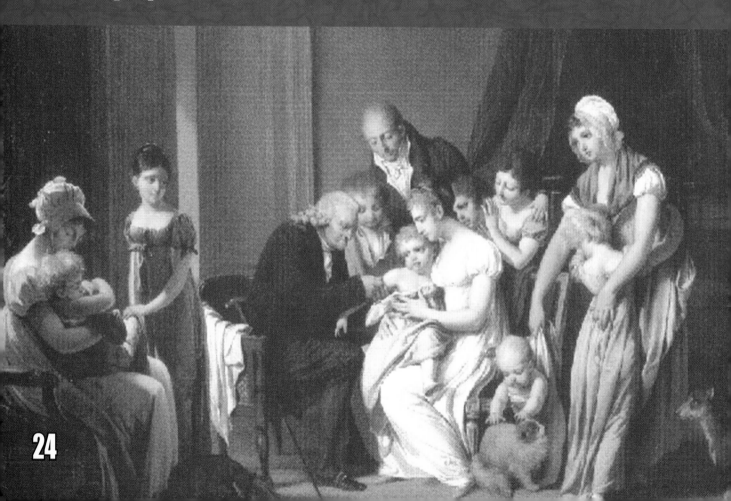

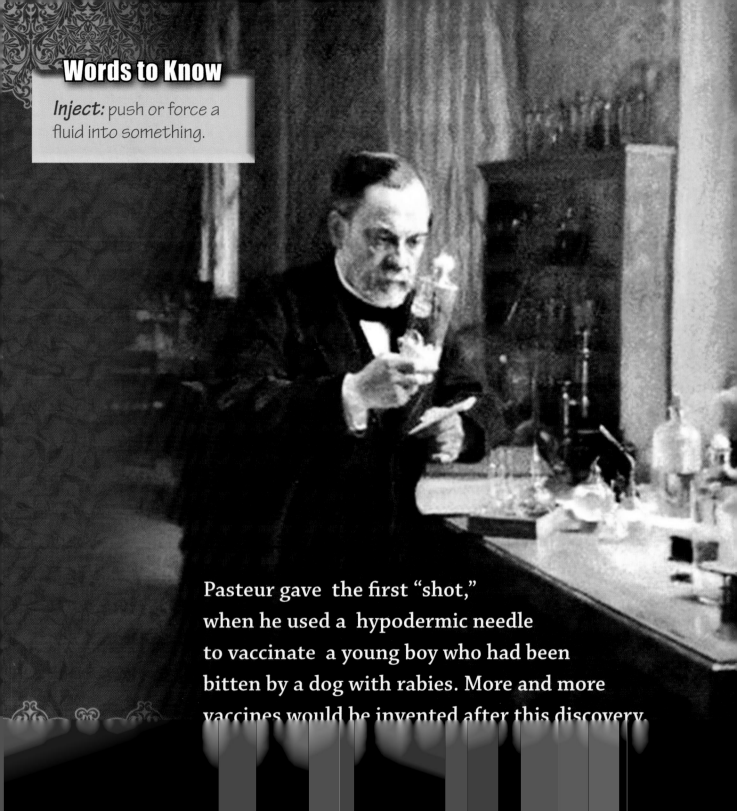

Pasteur gave the first "shot," when he used a hypodermic needle to vaccinate a young boy who had been bitten by a dog with rabies. More and more vaccines would be invented after this discovery.

POLIO

Polio is one of the oldest diseases in the world. It's been causing paralysis and death for most of human history. The stone engraving to the right shows an Egyptian boy with a leg withered from polio. The stone is over 3,000 years old!

By the 1920s, polio was one of the world's scariest diseases. People got sick with no warning—and there was no cure. Some people ended up having to be in "iron lungs" (shown on the page to the right) in order to breathe. Others were on crutches or in wheelchairs for the rest of their lives.

A man named Jonas Salk changed all that when he invented the first polio vaccine. Children lined up for the immunization—and parents breathed a sigh of relief that their children were finally safe from the mysterious and deadly disease.

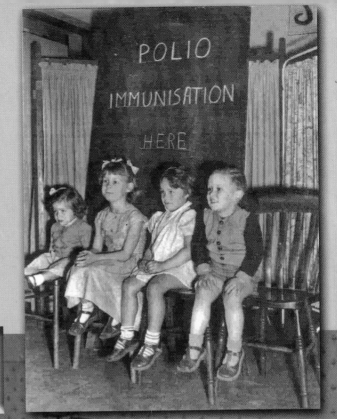

Words to Know

Paralysis: loss of the ability to move part or all of the body.

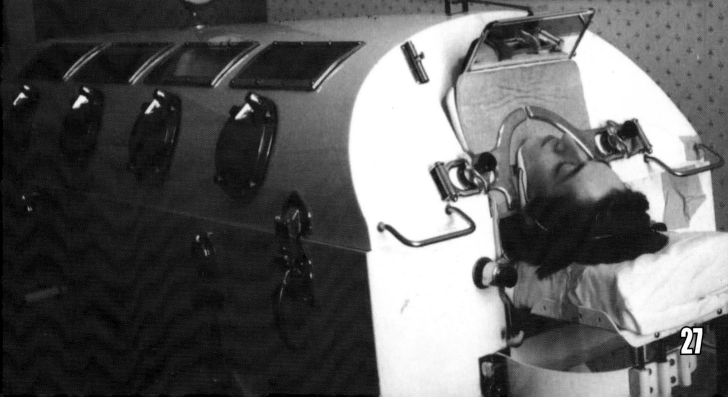

Whooping Cough

Whooping cough (also known as pertussis) is a respiratory disease caused by the bacteria shown on this page. When someone has whooping cough, thick mucus builds up in the lungs and clogs air passages, triggering violent coughing spells. The bacteria release poisons that can cause high fevers, convulsions, brain damage, and death.

In the United States in the early years of the 20th century, nearly 10,000 children a year died of whooping cough. Today, however, children in the U.S. are protected against this disease with vaccinations. In Africa and other poor regions of the world, where vaccinations are not always available, whooping cough is still the killer it once was.

Measles

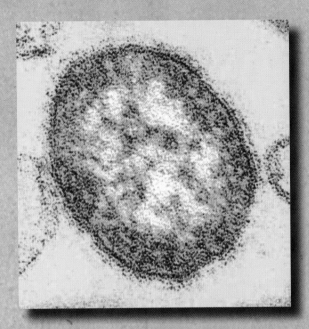

The itchy red rash shown here on the child's hand used to be an inevitable part of everyone's childhood. Caused by the virus shown above, measles has been nearly wiped out in the United States, Canada, and much of Europe, where most children are vaccinated against it. In the world's poorer nations, however, more than 17 million children get sick from this virus each year, and more than 200,000 of them die.

Mumps

Words to Know

Saliva: mix of water, protein, and salts that helps soften and break down food for digestion.

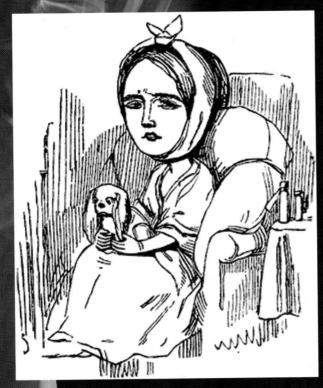

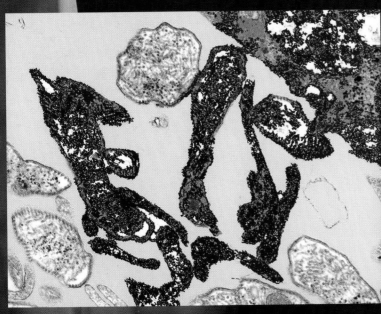

Mumps is caused by a virus (shown below) that usually spreads through saliva. It causes swelling and pain in the glands that make saliva, found toward the back of each cheek, between the ear and jaw (shown on the page to the left).

Mumps was another common childhood disease until 1967, when children began to be vaccinated against it. Since almost half of the world's nations still don't offer their children mumps vaccinations, outbreaks of mumps sometimes still occur in various parts of the world. Mumps is not dangerous for children—but it can be for an adult who catches it.

Tetanus

Also known as lockjaw, tetanus causes severe muscle contractions (as shown below) and ultimately, death. Vaccinations now protect us against the bacteria (right).

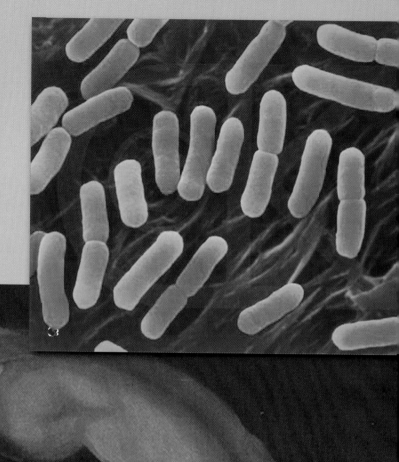

Meningitis

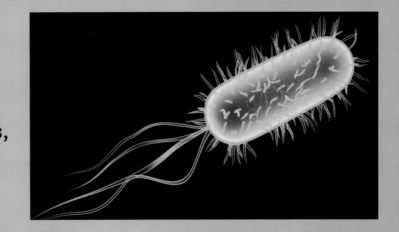

Meningitis causes the meninges, the lining of the brain, to become enflamed and swollen. Meningitis can cause brain damage and death. Several different germs, including the bacteria and the virus to the right, can produce meningitis—but a few meningitis vaccinations offer protection against many of the germs that can cause this disease.

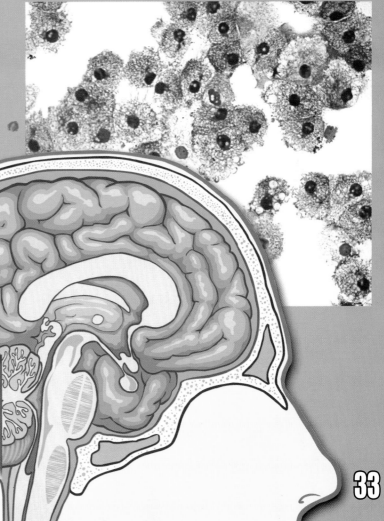

Words to Know

Inflammation: a response of body tissues to injury or disease, causing redness, swelling, and pain.

Chickenpox

The chickenpox virus causes red, itchy spots like the ones this child has. The vaccine that prevents chickenpox is one of the newest childhood immunizations.

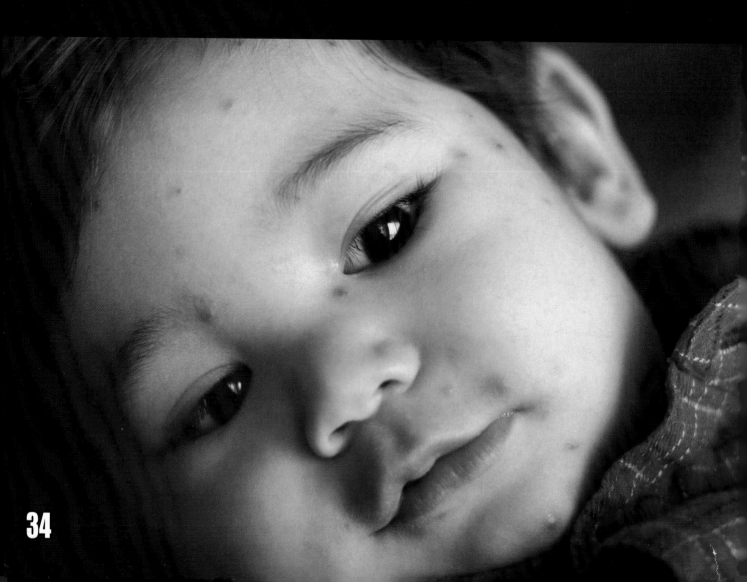

34

The Flu

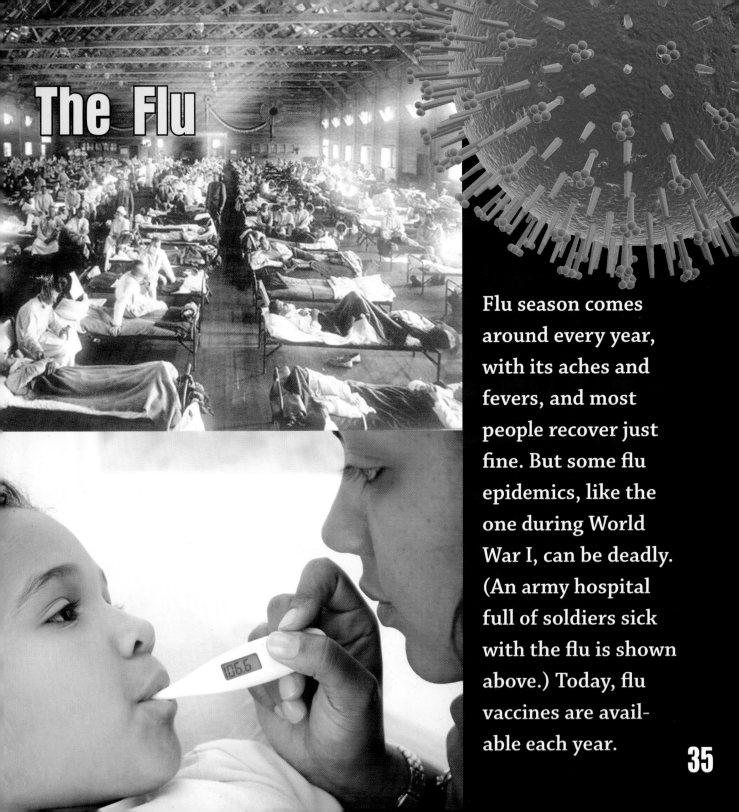

Flu season comes around every year, with its aches and fevers, and most people recover just fine. But some flu epidemics, like the one during World War I, can be deadly. (An army hospital full of soldiers sick with the flu is shown above.) Today, flu vaccines are available each year.

HPV

Human papillomavirus (HPV, shown to the right) can cause cervical cancer. Today, girls who receive the HPV vaccine are less apt to get this form of cancer.

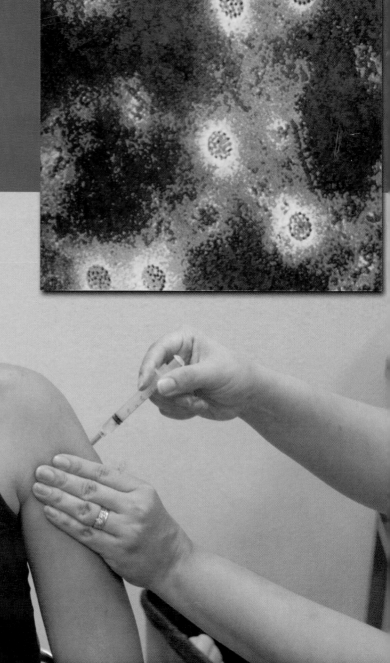

Other Diseases

Today, babies get shots for many sicknesses: hepatitis, diphtheria, and rotavirus are just a few. Each year, researchers develop new vaccines to protect against other diseases too.

Words to Know

Hepatitis: disease that causes inflammation of the liver.

Diphtheria: serious disease that produces a toxin (poison) that causes inflammation in the lining of the throat, nose, and windpipe.

Rotavirus: viruses that cause diarrhea in young children.

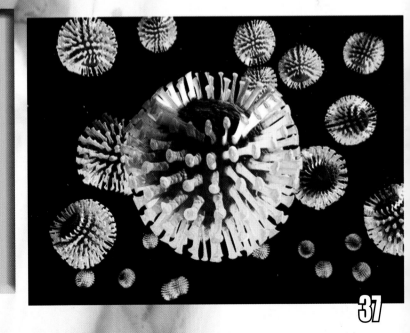

How Have Vaccines Changed the World?

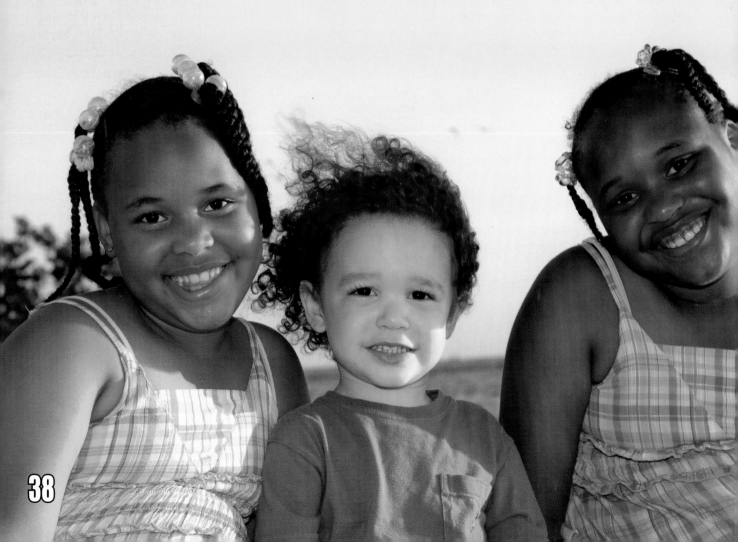

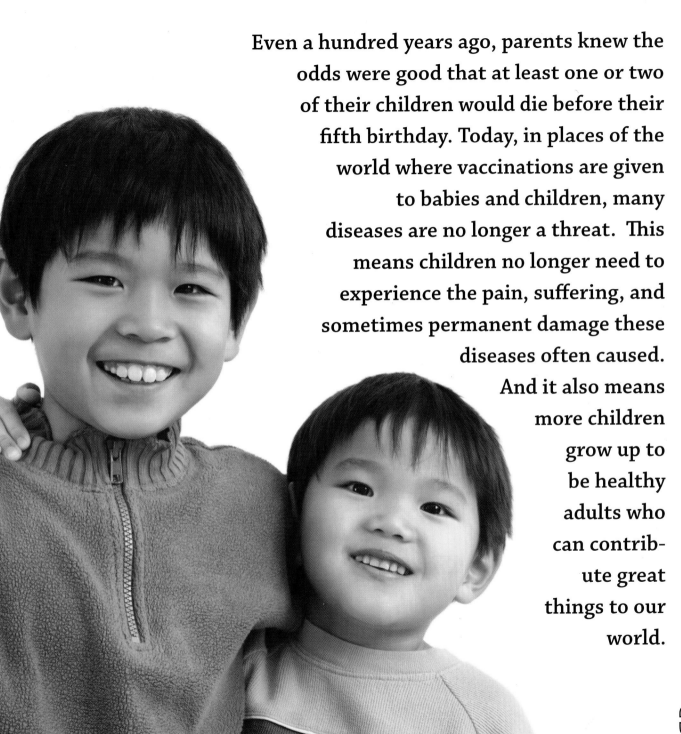

Even a hundred years ago, parents knew the odds were good that at least one or two of their children would die before their fifth birthday. Today, in places of the world where vaccinations are given to babies and children, many diseases are no longer a threat. This means children no longer need to experience the pain, suffering, and sometimes permanent damage these diseases often caused. And it also means more children grow up to be healthy adults who can contribute great things to our world.

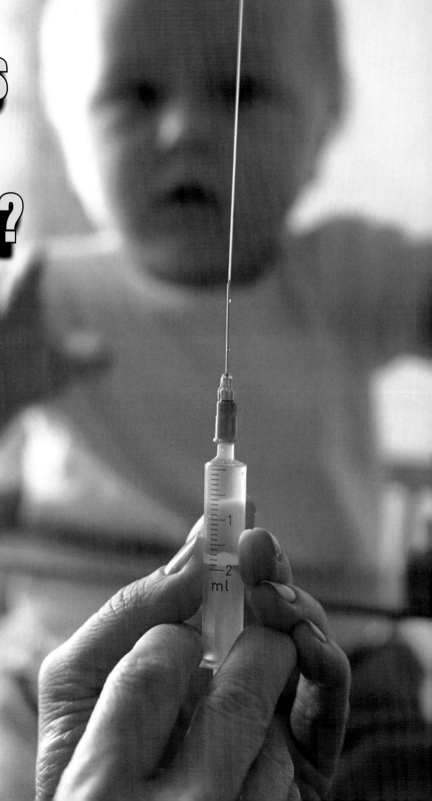

Who Needs to Be Vaccinated?

Doctors recommend that parents begin their babies' vaccinations soon after birth. These shots will continue through childhood. Booster shots may also be needed in adulthood.

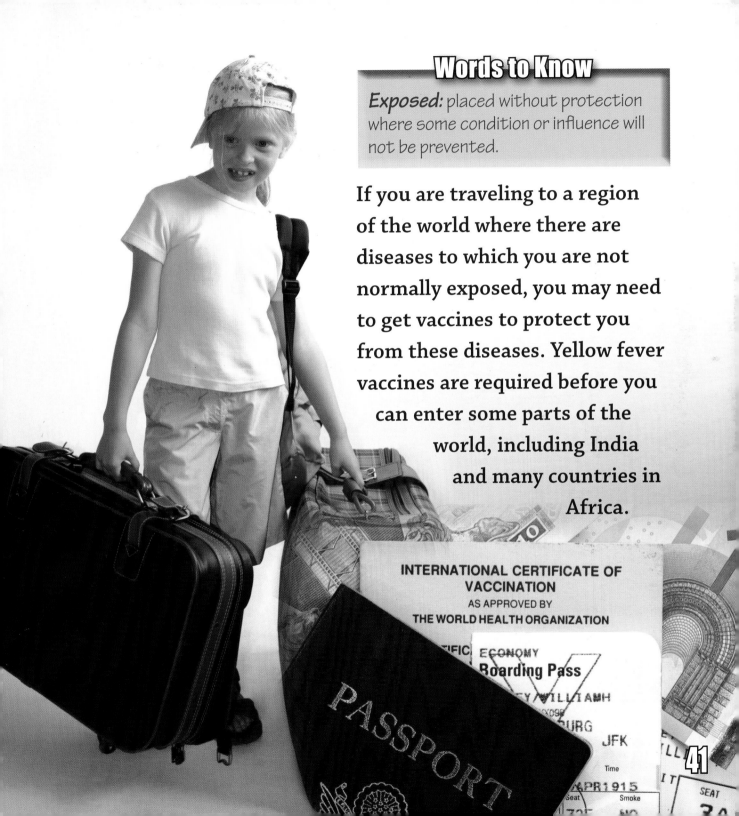

Exposed: placed without protection where some condition or influence will not be prevented.

If you are traveling to a region of the world where there are diseases to which you are not normally exposed, you may need to get vaccines to protect you from these diseases. Yellow fever vaccines are required before you can enter some parts of the world, including India and many countries in Africa.

INTERNATIONAL CERTIFICATE OF
VACCINATION
AS APPROVED BY
THE WORLD HEALTH ORGANIZATION

ECONOMY
Boarding Pass

PASSPORT

JFK

41

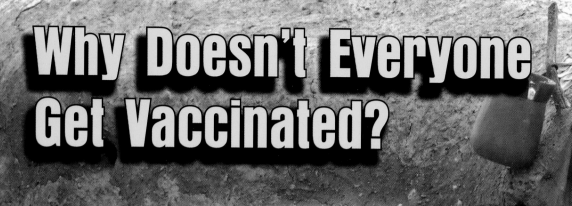

Why Doesn't Everyone Get Vaccinated?

Shots may be a part of growing up for children in some parts of the world—but for children in other parts of the world, including the African children shown here, shots may not even be available.

If everyone gets shots, won't the diseases eventually be wiped out?

A: Yes, you're right: the more children in a community who are vaccinated, the less likely it is that anyone, even those who have not been immunized, will get sick because there are fewer hosts for the germs that cause disease. Eventually, the disease will be wiped out altogether. Scientists believe that smallpox no longer exists anywhere except for in laboratories. Until doctors are sure a disease no longer exists, though, it is important to keep getting shots, since it only takes one person to carry a germ that starts an epidemic.

Each year in Africa, thousands of children die from diseases that no one worries about anymore in other parts of the world. In some parts of Africa, for example, a child dies of measles every minute. Mothers don't even bother to give their babies real names until the children have gotten measles and survived. Other children die of tetanus, diphtheria, whooping cough, polio, and yellow fever. All these children could have been saved if they had had the shots children in other parts of the world take for granted. These children may never have been to a doctor—so how can they get their shots? Their parents may have never even heard that immunizations exist that could save their children.

Sometimes people COULD have their children immunized, but they decide not to. The picture below is from the 1700s, and it shows the distrust some people felt about the cowpox fluids being used to vaccinate against smallpox. People didn't like the idea of putting "cow disease" inside them. Notice the little cows that the artist showed popping out of all these people who had been given Dr. Jenner's vaccine.

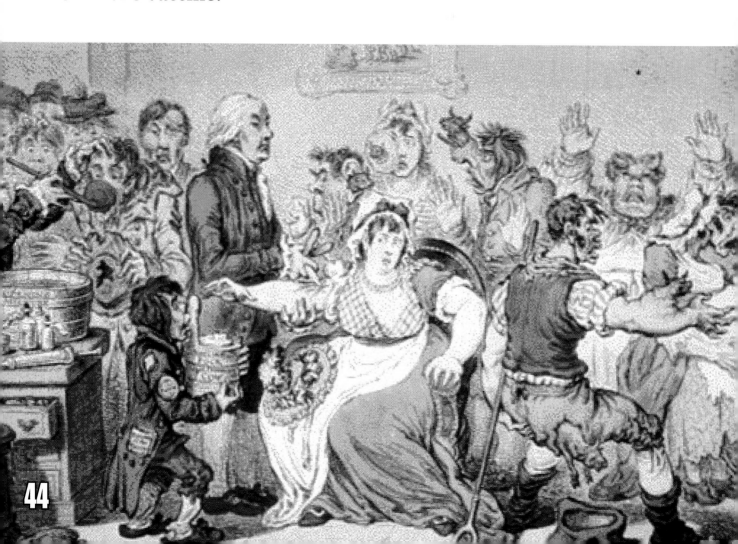

Today, people also have doubts about the safety of vaccinations given to children, and some parents are choosing not to have their children vaccinated. These parents worry that the vaccines may have harmful side effects.

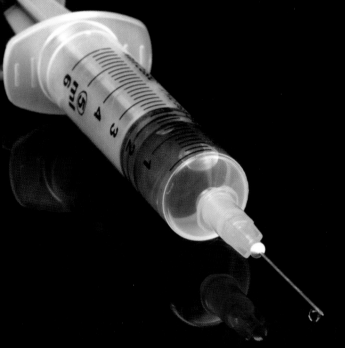

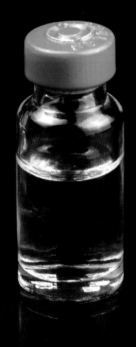

Did You Know?

Autism is a brain disorder that begins in early childhood and continues through adulthood, affecting a person's ability to communicate and interact with others.

Some people think that there may be a connection between the rise of autism and the shots children are routinely given. Most doctors, however, disagree. They say that the protection shots offer against diseases far outweighs their risks.

What Is the World Doing?

The World Health Organization (WHO) is the part of the United Nations (UN) that deals with health issues. (The headquarters in Geneva, Switzerland are shown below.)

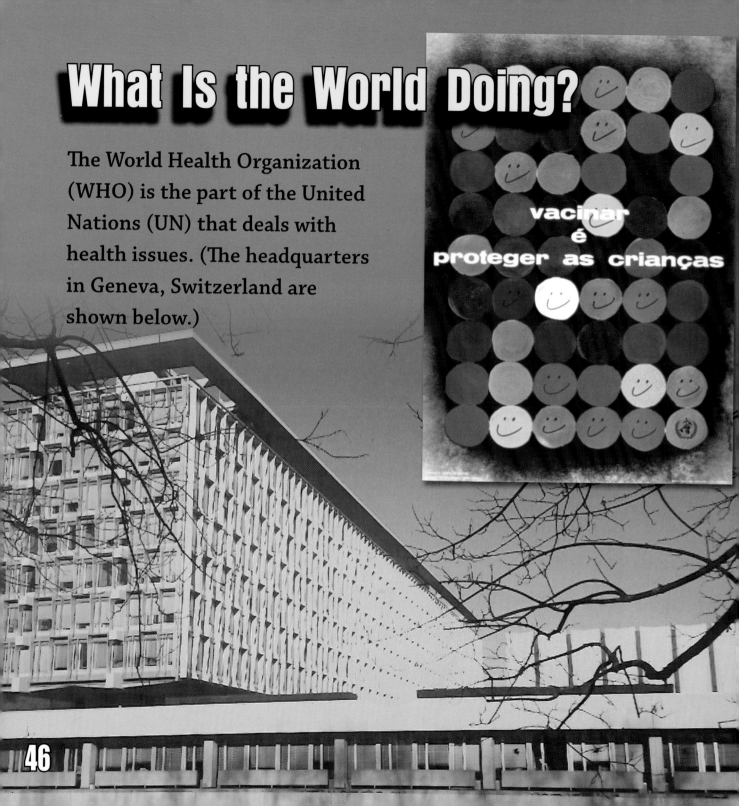

vacinar
é
proteger as crianças

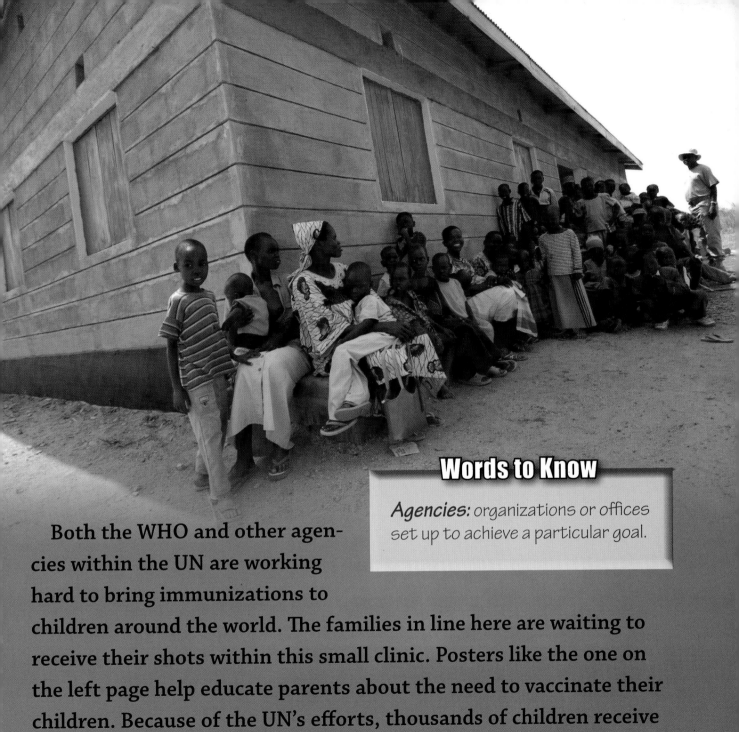

Both the WHO and other agencies within the UN are working hard to bring immunizations to children around the world. The families in line here are waiting to receive their shots within this small clinic. Posters like the one on the left page help educate parents about the need to vaccinate their children. Because of the UN's efforts, thousands of children receive life-saving vaccinations each year.

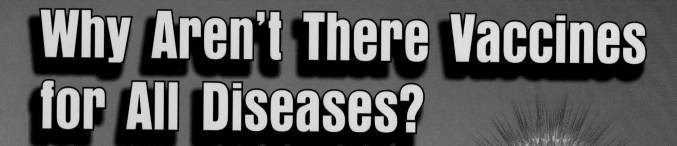

Why Aren't There Vaccines for All Diseases?

Since vaccinations keep a person from ever getting a particular disease, you'd think that by now doctors would be immunizing people against all diseases. It seems like the same principle of giving a weak or dead version of the germ would work for all diseases, right?

Unfortunately, the answer to that question is, "Wrong." The reason why some diseases—like the common cold for instance—don't have a vaccine is because the germs (the viruses and bacteria) that cause them keep changing. The genetic material inside the germs is constantly mutating, which means that each new generation of germs is slightly different from the one before. You could build up antibodies against the old version—but it wouldn't do you any good when the new version invaded your body. Your antibodies wouldn't recognize it.

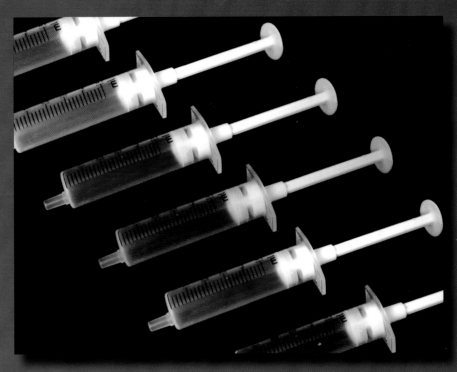

Words to Know

Genetic: having to do with genes, the material that is passed down from parents to offspring.

Mutating: making changes to the genes.

49

What Are Scientists Doing?

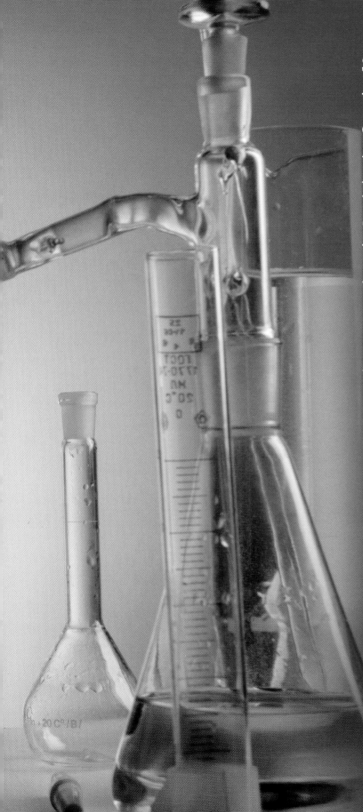

Scientists are working hard to find new vaccines for more diseases. They are looking for the right substances that will help us build immunity against each enemy that invades our bodies. Some of these trial vaccines can be tested on animals, to see if they work. Others, however, may need to be tried out on humans. This is another reason why scientists may not yet have developed a vaccine for a particular disease: for moral reasons, they cannot do research that might harm human beings. This means they must try to reproduce conditions in test tubes and petri dishes to make sure a possible vaccine is absolutely safe before it is tested on people. Research is a slow job!

51

Why Do Vaccines Have to Hurt?

Lots of people—childen AND adults—are afraid of shots. Some people are so afraid that they feel shaky or even faint. It's not because shots really hurt all that much (after all, they're really just a prick that only takes a second). But being scared isn't always about what makes sense. Some people just find shots scary. They wonder why scientists can't invent another way of getting that weak or dead germ inside them.

Actually, not all vaccines do hurt. Some immunizations can be given orally—through your mouth. The newer polio vaccine is an example of an oral immunization. You usually swallow the vaccine on a sugar cube or in a small, sweet swallow of syrupy liquid.

These vaccines are made of living germs. They can't usually survive the acids in your stomach, but they get into the lining of your mouth and nose enough to trigger your body to make antibodies—but not enough to make you sick. The problem with giving someone live germs is there's a chance they will make people sick with the actual disease.

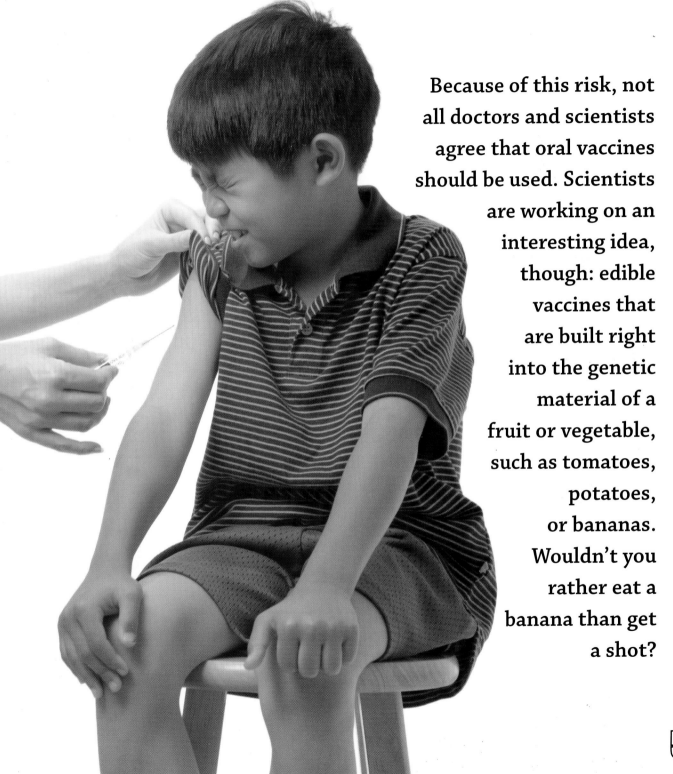

Because of this risk, not all doctors and scientists agree that oral vaccines should be used. Scientists are working on an interesting idea, though: edible vaccines that are built right into the genetic material of a fruit or vegetable, such as tomatoes, potatoes, or bananas. Wouldn't you rather eat a banana than get a shot?

53

Why Do I Need to Get Booster Shots?

It's bad enough getting shots in the first place. Having to go back every few years for more shots can seem like pure torture. Unfortunately, just one shot is seldom enough to make you immune against a particular disease.

Whenever you're vaccinated, your immune system activates a certain number of special cells called B-cells. These B-cells will multiply and some of them will make temporary antibodies. Others of these multiplying B-cells will become something scientists call "memory cells." Memory B-cells can last for years and years in our bodies and are able to make antibodies whenever the germ you were vaccinated against infects your body.

Words to Know

Activates: sets in motion, makes active.

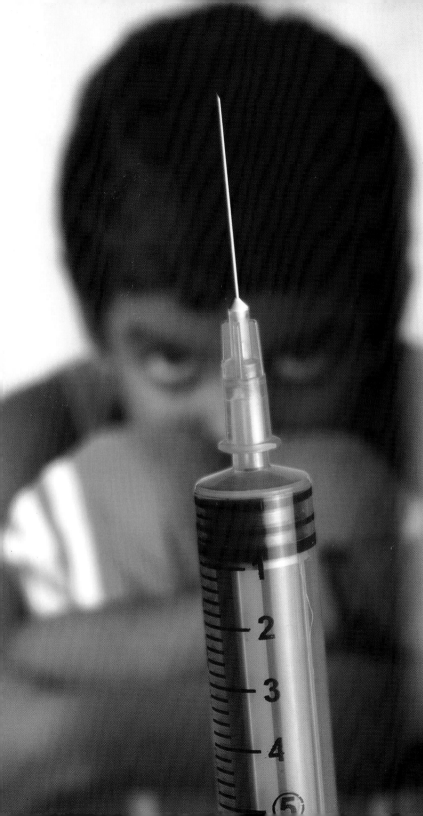

But the first vaccine doesn't get enough of the B-cells activated. Booster shots activate more B-cells. When more B-cells are activated, more antibodies are made. More antibodies mean more invading germs will be surrounded and destroyed.

In other words, your booster shots make sure you can completely fight off a particular germ—so you never have to worry about it again.

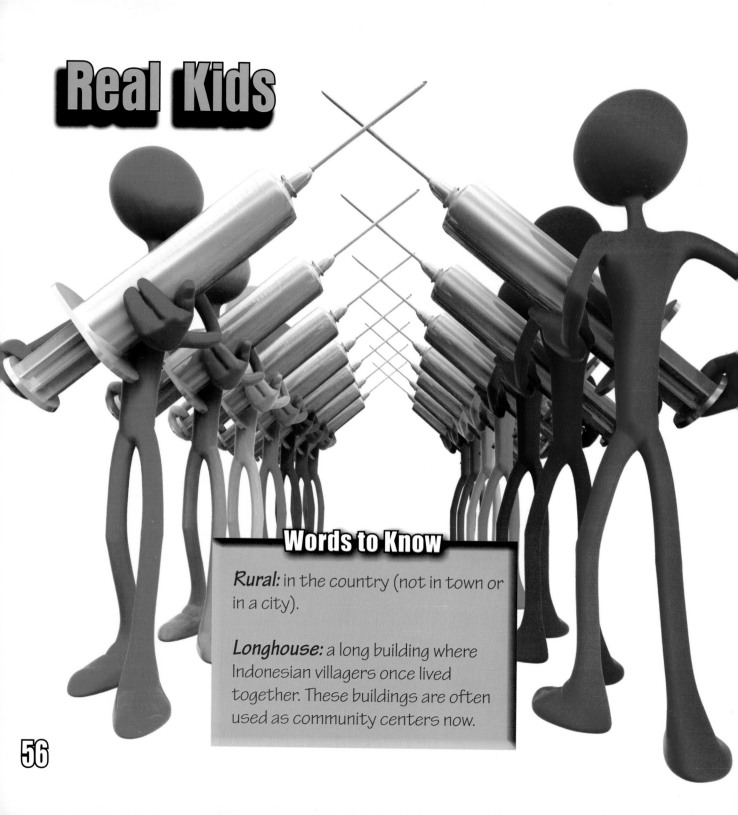

Real Kids

Words to Know

Rural: in the country (not in town or in a city).

Longhouse: a long building where Indonesian villagers once lived together. These buildings are often used as community centers now.

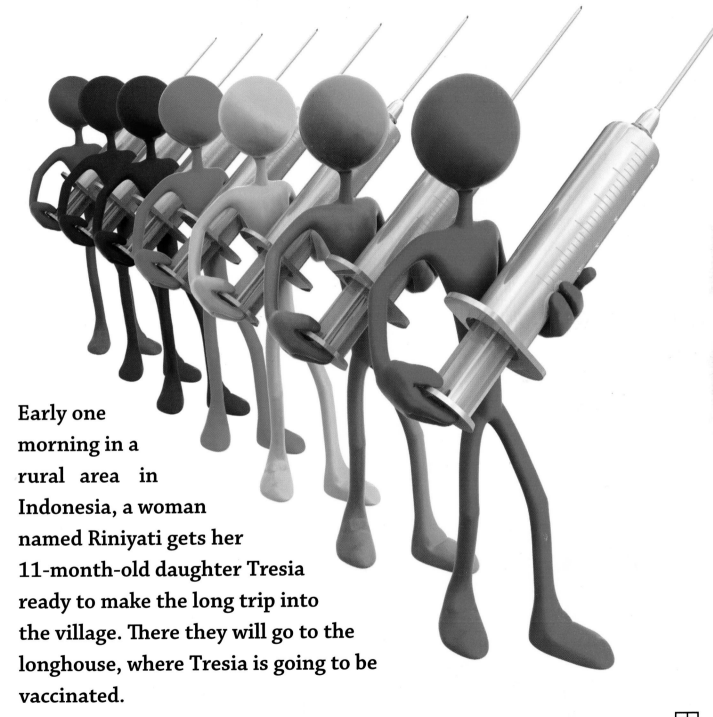

Early one morning in a rural area in Indonesia, a woman named Riniyati gets her 11-month-old daughter Tresia ready to make the long trip into the village. There they will go to the longhouse, where Tresia is going to be vaccinated.

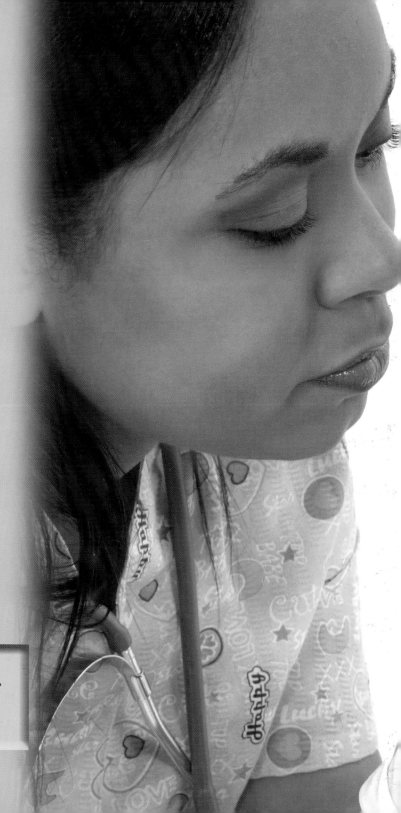

It's a long walk to the village for Riniyati, but she knows it's worth it. "I heard that measles and polio could hurt my child and she could even die if I didn't get her immunized," she told UN workers.

Getting the vaccines to remote places like Riniyati's village is hard work for UN workers as well. The vaccines Tresia will receive were flown from a factory in Java, then shipped by truck to health offices. From there, the vaccines went by boat.

Words to Know

Remote: far away from any city or transportation route.

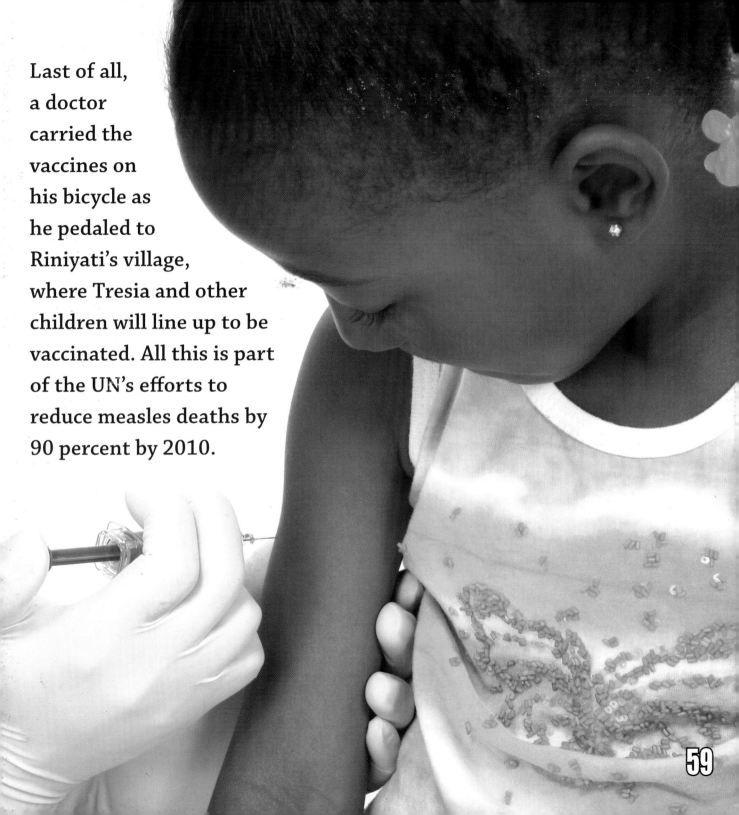

Last of all, a doctor carried the vaccines on his bicycle as he pedaled to Riniyati's village, where Tresia and other children will line up to be vaccinated. All this is part of the UN's efforts to reduce measles deaths by 90 percent by 2010.

Find Out More

These Web sites will tell you more about immunizations and the history of some of the diseases they protect against.

CDC's Vaccines and Immunizations
www.cdc.gov/vaccines

Kid's Health: Polio
www.kidshealth.org/parent/ infections/bacterial_viral/polio.html

Mayo Clinic: Immunizations
www.mayoclinic.com/health/vaccines/CC00014

MedlinePlus: Vaccines
0-www.nlm.nih.gov.catalog.llu.edu/ medlineplus/immunization.
html

NHS Immunisations
www.immunisation.nhs.uk

Teen's Health: Immunizations
kidshealth.org/teen/school_jobs/college/immunizations.html

WHO Immunizations
www.who.int/topics/immunization/en

WHO Smallpox
www.who.int/mediacentre/factsheets/smallpox/en

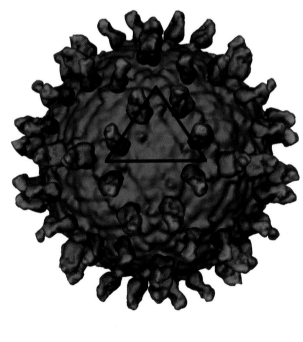
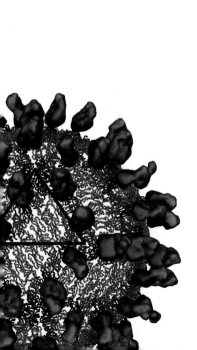
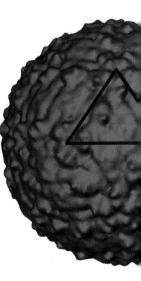

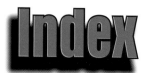

Index

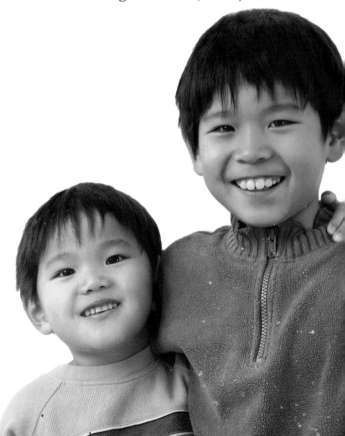

Picture Credits

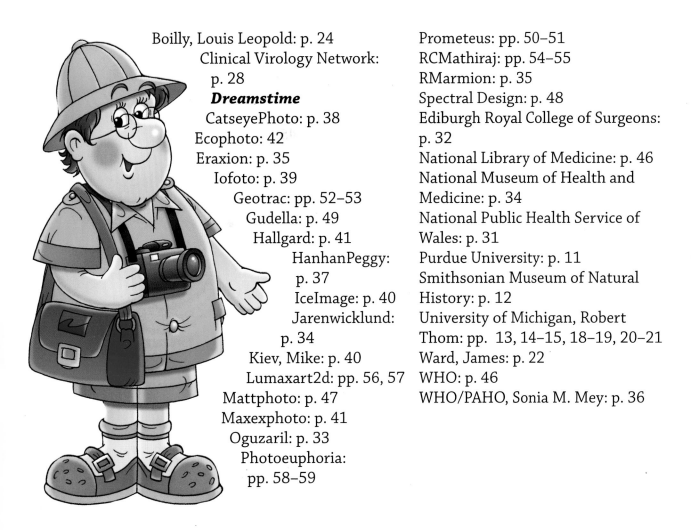

Boilly, Louis Leopold: p. 24
Clinical Virology Network: p. 28
Dreamstime
CatseyePhoto: p. 38
Ecophoto: 42
Eraxion: p. 35
Iofoto: p. 39
Geotrac: pp. 52–53
Gudella: p. 49
Hallgard: p. 41
HanhanPeggy: p. 37
IceImage: p. 40
Jarenwicklund: p. 34
Kiev, Mike: p. 40
Lumaxart2d: pp. 56, 57
Mattphoto: p. 47
Maxexphoto: p. 41
Oguzaril: p. 33
Photoeuphoria: pp. 58–59

Prometeus: pp. 50–51
RCMathiraj: pp. 54–55
RMarmion: p. 35
Spectral Design: p. 48
Ediburgh Royal College of Surgeons: p. 32
National Library of Medicine: p. 46
National Museum of Health and Medicine: p. 34
National Public Health Service of Wales: p. 31
Purdue University: p. 11
Smithsonian Museum of Natural History: p. 12
University of Michigan, Robert Thom: pp. 13, 14–15, 18–19, 20–21
Ward, James: p. 22
WHO: p. 46
WHO/PAHO, Sonia M. Mey: p. 36

About the Author

Rae Simons has written many books for young adults and children. She lives with her family in New York State in the U.S.

About the Consultant

Elise DeVore Berlan, MD, MPH, FAAP, is a faculty member of the Division of Adolescent Health at Nationwide Children's Hospital and an Assistant Professor of Clinical Pediatrics at The Ohio State University College of Medicine. She completed her Fellowship in Adolescent Medicine at Children's Hospital Boston and obtained a Master's Degree in Public Health at the Harvard School of Public Health. Dr. Berlan completed her residency in pediatrics at the Children's Hospital of Philadelphia, where she also served an additional year as Chief Resident. She received her medical degree from the University of Iowa College of Medicine.